# The Essential Guide to Intermittent Fasting for Women

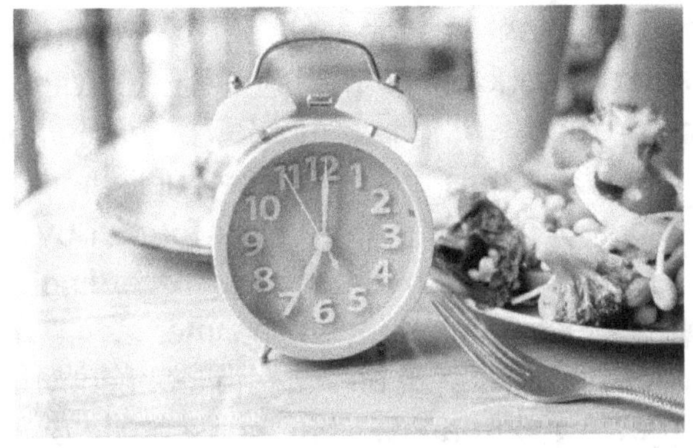

The Ultimate Ways to Lose Weight, Balance your Hormones, Transform your Body and Reset your Metabolism

Isaac Hendricks

# Table of Contents

# INTRODUCTION

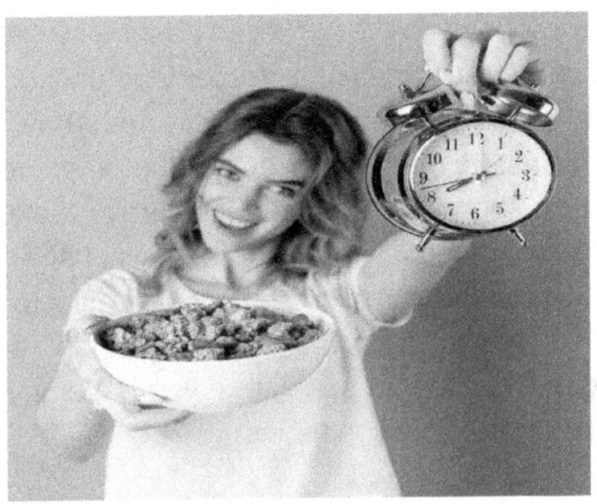

## What is Intermittent Fasting?

Intermittent fasting has gained immense popularity in recent years as a weight loss and wellness strategy. While it's true that intermittent fasting can benefit both men and women, there are some unique considerations for women who are considering embarking on this lifestyle change. In this essential guide to intermittent fasting for women, we'll explore the benefits, challenges, and best practices for women who want to incorporate intermittent fasting into their daily routines.

Intermittent fasting is a dietary pattern that cycles between periods of voluntary fasting and periods of eating. It does not prescribe which things to eat, but rather when to take them. The most popular methods of intermittent fasting include the 16:8 method (fasting for 16 hours and eating during an 8-hour window), the 5:2 method (fasting for two non-consecutive days of the week and eating normally for the other five), and alternate-day fasting (fasting every other day). Intermittent fasting has been shown to have potential health benefits, such as weight loss, improved insulin sensitivity, and reduced inflammation, but it's essential to consult a healthcare provider before starting any new dietary pattern, especially if you have any underlying medical conditions.

One of the most significant benefits of intermittent fasting for women is its potential to support healthy hormone levels. Women's hormonal cycles can be complex and sometimes unpredictable, making it challenging to maintain a consistent weight or manage symptoms like bloating or cramps. Intermittent fasting has been shown to help regulate oestrogen levels, which can improve symptoms like mood swings, breast tenderness, and menstrual cramps. Additionally, intermittent fasting may help reduce insulin resistance, which can contribute to weight gain and hormonal imbalances.

Another benefit of intermittent fasting for women is its potential to support healthy ageing. As we age, our bodies become less efficient at processing glucose (sugar) and regulating insulin levels. This can lead to age-related diseases like type 2 diabetes and Alzheimer's disease. Intermittent fasting has been shown to help improve insulin sensitivity, which can reduce the risk of these age-related diseases and promote healthy ageing.

However, there are also some unique challenges that women may face when embarking on an intermittent fasting journey. One of the most significant challenges is managing hunger and cravings during the fasting periods. Women may be more susceptible to hunger due to hormonal fluctuations or other factors like pregnancy or breastfeeding. It's essential to find strategies that work for you, such as drinking plenty of water or herbal tea during the fasting period or incorporating healthy fats like avocado or nuts into your meals during the eating periods to help keep you feeling fuller for longer.

Another challenge that women may face is managing menstrual cycles while intermittent fasting. Some women may experience changes in appetite or energy levels during their menstrual cycles, making it challenging to stick to a consistent intermittent fasting routine. It's essential to listen to your body and adjust your routine as needed during your menstrual cycle. This may mean shortening your fasting periods or adjusting your meal times to better align with your body's needs during this time.

In terms of best practices for women who want to incorporate intermittent fasting into their daily routines, there are a few key tips to consider:

**1. Start slow:** If you're new to intermittent fasting, it's essential to start slowly and gradually increase the length of your fasting periods over time. This will help your body adjust to the new routine and reduce the risk of any negative side effects like dizziness or fatigue.

**2. Listen to your body:** As mentioned earlier, it's essential to listen to your body and adjust your routine as needed during your menstrual cycle or other times when you may be experiencing changes in appetite or energy levels. Don't be too hard on yourself if you need to make adjustments - the goal is to find a routine that works best for you!

**3. Focus on whole foods:** When you are eating during your designated window, focus on consuming whole foods like fruits, vegetables, whole grains, and lean proteins instead of processed foods or sugary snacks. This will help provide your body with the nutrients it needs while also supporting healthy weight loss goals.

**4. Stay hydrated:** Drinking plenty of water throughout the day is essential for maintaining good health and supporting weight loss goals through intermittent fasting. Make an effort to drink at least 8-10 glasses of water per day!

**5. Consult with a healthcare professional:** If you have any underlying health conditions or concerns about starting an intermittent fasting routine, it's essential to consult with a healthcare professional before getting started. They can provide personalised guidance based on your individual needs and help ensure that you're following a safe and effective routine!

## Why should women consider intermittent fasting?

While Intermittent fasting (IF) is traditionally associated with weight loss, IF has gained popularity among women for its numerous health benefits. Here are some reasons why women should consider incorporating IF into their lifestyle:

### Promotes weight loss:

IF can help women achieve their weight loss goals by reducing calorie intake. Studies have shown that women who follow IF lose more weight than those who follow traditional calorie-restricted diets.

### Regulates hormones:

IF can help regulate hormones such as insulin, leptin, and ghrelin, which are crucial for weight management and overall health. This can lead to improved metabolism, reduced inflammation, and lower risk of chronic diseases such as diabetes and heart disease.

## Enhances cognitive function:

IF has been shown to improve cognitive function, including memory, focus, and concentration. This is due to the fact that fasting promotes the production of brain-derived neurotrophic factor (BDNF), a protein that supports the growth and survival of neurons in the brain.

## Reduces oxidative stress:

IF can help reduce oxidative stress, which is a major contributor to aging and chronic diseases such as cancer and Alzheimer's disease. This is because fasting activates cellular repair mechanisms that help combat oxidative stress.

## Improves insulin sensitivity:

IF can improve insulin sensitivity, which is crucial for managing blood sugar levels and preventing type 2 diabetes. This is because fasting helps the body become more efficient at using insulin to transport glucose into cells where it can be used for energy.

## Boosts energy levels:

Contrary to popular belief, IF can actually boost energy levels by promoting the production of ketones, which are a source of fuel for the brain and body during fasting. This can lead to improved mental clarity and physical performance during workouts.


Enhances longevity:

IF has been shown to promote longevity by activating cellular repair mechanisms that help combat aging at the cellular level. This is because fasting helps the body enter a state of autophagy, which is a process by which cells recycle and remove damaged components.

In conclusion, IF offers numerous health benefits for women, including weight loss, hormone regulation, cognitive function enhancement, reduced oxidative stress, improved insulin sensitivity, boosted energy levels, and enhanced longevity. Women who are interested in incorporating IF into their lifestyle should consult with a healthcare provider or a registered dietitian to ensure it is safe and appropriate for their individual needs.

## How does intermittent fasting differ for women?

Intermittent fasting (IF) is a dietary pattern that involves alternating periods of fasting and eating. While the basic principles of IF are the same for both men and women, there are some differences in how it affects women's bodies due to hormonal fluctuations.

- Menstrual cycle: Women's menstrual cycles can impact how they respond to IF. During menstruation, oestrogen and progesterone levels are low, which can make it easier for women to fast. However, during ovulation and the luteal phase, these hormones increase, which can make it more challenging for women to stick to a strict fasting schedule.

- Hormonal fluctuations: Women's hormonal fluctuations also affect how their bodies respond to IF. During menstruation, oestrogen and progesterone levels are low, which can lead to a decrease in appetite. However, during ovulation and the luteal phase, these hormones increase, which can lead to an increase in appetite and cravings. This can make it more challenging for women to stick to a strict fasting schedule during these times.

- Nutrient needs: Women's nutrient needs are different from men's due to differences in body composition and hormonal fluctuations. Because of menstrual blood loss, women require more iron than men. During IF, women may need to pay closer attention to their nutrient intake to ensure they are meeting their needs.

- Pregnancy and breastfeeding: Women who are pregnant or breastfeeding should consult with a healthcare provider before starting IF as it may not be appropriate during these times due to the increased nutrient needs of both mother and baby.

- Mental health: Women may also experience different mental health effects from IF than men due to hormonal fluctuations. For example, during ovulation and the luteal phase, women may experience mood swings and increased stress levels, which could impact how they respond to IF.

In summary, while the basic principles of IF are the same for both men and women, women's hormonal fluctuations can impact how they respond to IF. Women should pay close attention to their nutrient needs and consult with a healthcare provider if they are pregnant or breastfeeding before starting IF. Additionally, women may need to adjust their fasting schedule based on their menstrual cycle and hormonal fluctuations.

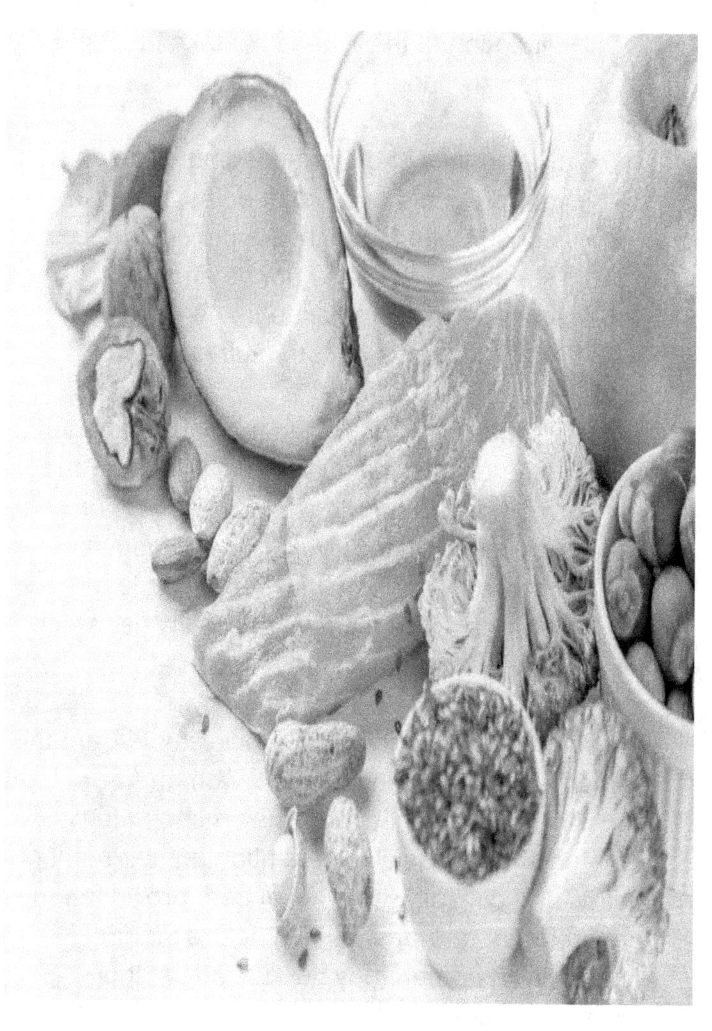

# CHAPTER ONE

## Benefits of Intermittent Fasting for Women

### Weight loss and body composition changes

Intermittent fasting (IF) has gained popularity in recent years as a weight loss and overall health strategy. While both men and women can benefit from IF, studies have shown that women may experience unique benefits, particularly in terms of weight loss and body composition changes.

### Weight Loss:

One of the most significant benefits of IF for women is its potential for weight loss. A study published in the Journal of Translational Medicine found that women who practised IF lost more weight than those who followed a traditional calorie-restricted diet. The study also found that women who followed IF experienced a greater reduction in body fat percentage than those on the calorie-restricted diet.

The reason for this may be due to the fact that IF can help regulate hormones such as insulin and cortisol, which are known to contribute to weight gain. By reducing insulin levels, IF can promote fat burning and prevent the storage of excess calories as fat. Additionally, IF can help reduce cortisol levels, which is a stress hormone that can lead to weight gain around the midsection.

## Body Composition Changes:

In addition to weight loss, IF has been shown to result in significant body composition changes for women. A study published in the Journal of Obesity found that women who followed IF experienced a greater increase in lean body mass (LBM) than those on a traditional calorie-restricted diet. LBM refers to the amount of muscle, bone, and other non-fat tissue in the body.

The increase in LBM is important because it helps to improve overall body composition by reducing the amount of fat tissue while preserving muscle mass. This is particularly important for women as they age, as muscle mass tends to decrease with age, leading to a loss of strength and mobility. By preserving muscle mass through IF, women can help maintain their overall health and wellbeing as they age.

Another study published in the Journal of Nutrition & Metabolism found that women who followed IF experienced a significant reduction in waist circumference, which is a measure of abdominal fat. This is important because excess abdominal fat has been linked to an increased risk of chronic diseases such as diabetes, heart disease, and certain types of cancer. By reducing abdominal fat through IF, women can help improve their overall health and reduce their risk of these diseases.

Conclusion:

In conclusion, intermittent fasting offers unique benefits for women, particularly in terms of weight loss and body composition changes. By promoting fat burning, preserving muscle mass, and reducing abdominal fat, IF can help improve overall health and wellbeing for women. However, it's important to note that individual results may vary and it's always recommended to consult with a healthcare professional before starting any new diet or exercise program.

## Improved metabolic health and insulin sensitivity

Intermittent fasting (IF) has gained popularity in recent years as a weight loss and health promotion strategy. While the benefits of IF have been studied in both men and women, research suggests that women may experience unique advantages, particularly in terms of improved metabolic health and insulin sensitivity.

Metabolic health refers to the body's ability to efficiently process nutrients and maintain stable blood sugar levels. Insulin sensitivity, on the other hand, describes how well the body responds to insulin, the hormone that regulates blood sugar levels. Poor metabolic health and insulin resistance are risk factors for chronic diseases such as type 2 diabetes, cardiovascular disease, and obesity.

Several studies have shown that IF can improve metabolic health and insulin sensitivity in women. A 2019 systematic review and meta-analysis of 13 randomised controlled trials found that IF led to significant reductions in fasting blood sugar, insulin, and triglyceride levels in women, as well as improvements in insulin sensitivity

Another study published in the Journal of Translational Medicine found that women who followed a 16:8 IF regimen for 12 weeks experienced significant reductions in body weight, body fat percentage, and waist circumference, as well as improvements in insulin sensitivity

The mechanisms behind these benefits are not fully understood, but some theories suggest that IF may help to reduce inflammation, oxidative stress, and insulin resistance

During periods of fasting, the body may also activate cellular processes such as autophagy, which involves the removal of damaged cell components and may help to prevent cellular dysfunction and disease

It's important to note that while IF can be beneficial for many women, it's not suitable for everyone. Women who are pregnant or breastfeeding should avoid IF due to the potential risks to foetal development and infant growth

Women with a history of eating disorders or disordered eating patterns should also approach IF with caution and seek guidance from a healthcare provider or registered dietitian.

In conclusion, intermittent fasting can lead to improved metabolic health and insulin sensitivity in women. While more research is needed to fully understand the mechanisms behind these benefits, it's clear that IF can be a safe and effective strategy for promoting overall health and wellness in women. As with any dietary or lifestyle intervention, it's important to approach IF with caution and seek guidance from a healthcare provider or registered dietitian to ensure that it's appropriate for your individual needs and goals.

## Reduced inflammation and oxidative stress

Intermittent fasting (IF) has gained popularity in recent years as a dietary pattern that involves alternating periods of fasting and eating. While the benefits of IF have been widely studied, particularly in men, research has also shown that women can experience significant health benefits from this dietary approach. In this article, we will explore the role of reduced inflammation and oxidative stress in the benefits of IF for women.

Inflammation is the body's natural response to damage or infection. However, chronic inflammation has been linked to various diseases such as cancer, cardiovascular disease, and Alzheimer's disease. IF has been found to reduce inflammation in both men and women. A study published in the Journal of Translational Medicine found that women who followed an IF regimen for 12 weeks had significantly lower levels of inflammatory markers such as C-reactive protein (CRP) and interleukin-6 (IL-6) compared to a control group.

Oxidative stress is a condition that occurs when there is an imbalance between the production of free radicals and the body's ability to detoxify them. Free radicals are unstable chemicals that can cause cell damage and contribute to the ageing and disease process. IF has been found to reduce oxidative stress in both men and women. A study published in the Journal of Nutrition found that women who followed an IF regimen for 12 weeks had significantly lower levels of oxidative stress markers such as malondialdehyde (MDA) and 8-isoprostane compared to a control group.

The mechanisms behind the anti-inflammatory and antioxidant effects of IF are not fully understood, but some theories have been proposed. One theory suggests that IF leads to a reduction in insulin levels, which in turn reduces inflammation and oxidative stress.
Another theory suggests that IF activates autophagy, a process by which cells remove damaged components, which reduces inflammation and oxidative stress.

In addition to reducing inflammation and oxidative stress, IF has also been found to improve other health outcomes in women. A study published in the Journal of Women's Health found that women who followed an IF regimen for 12 weeks had significant improvements in body composition, including a decrease in body fat percentage and a rise in lean body mass.
Another study published in the Journal of Obesity found that women who followed an IF regimen for 12 weeks had significant improvements in lipid profiles, including a decrease in triglycerides as well as a rise in HDL cholesterol.

In conclusion, reduced inflammation and oxidative stress are important benefits of intermittent fasting for women. The anti-inflammatory and antioxidant effects of IF may contribute to improved health outcomes such as improved body composition, lipid profiles, and reduced risk of chronic diseases. Further research is needed to fully understand the mechanisms behind these effects and to determine the optimal frequency, duration, and type of IF for women. However, these findings suggest that IF may be a promising dietary approach for promoting health and wellness in women.

## Enhanced cognitive function and brain health

Intermittent fasting (IF) has gained immense popularity in recent years as a weight loss and overall health strategy. However, beyond its weight loss benefits, research has shown that IF can also have significant positive effects on cognitive function and brain health, particularly for women.

### Cognitive Function:

Cognitive function refers to the mental processes involved in acquiring, retaining, and using knowledge and skills. IF has been found to improve cognitive function in women through several mechanisms.

Firstly, IF can increase levels of brain-derived neurotrophic factor (BDNF), a protein that plays a crucial role in the growth and survival of neurons in the brain. BDNF is essential for learning, memory, and cognitive function. Studies have shown that women who practise IF have higher levels of BDNF than those who do not fast.

Secondly, IF can reduce inflammation in the body, which is known to contribute to cognitive decline. Chronic inflammation can lead to oxidative stress and damage to brain cells, leading to cognitive impairment. By reducing inflammation, IF may help prevent or slow down cognitive decline in women.

Thirdly, IF can improve insulin sensitivity, which is linked to better cognitive function. Insulin resistance has been associated with cognitive impairment and dementia. By improving insulin sensitivity, IF may help prevent or delay cognitive decline in women.

Brain Health:

Brain health refers to the overall health and well-being of the brain. IF has been found to have several benefits for brain health in women.

Firstly, IF can reduce the risk of neurodegenerative diseases such as Alzheimer's and Parkinson's disease. These diseases are characterised by the accumulation of abnormal proteins in the brain, leading to cell death and cognitive decline. By reducing inflammation and oxidative stress, IF may help prevent or slow down the progression of these diseases in women.

Secondly, IF can improve memory and concentration in women. Studies have shown that women who practise IF have better memory and concentration than those who do not fast. This may be due to the increased levels of BDNF and improved insulin sensitivity associated with IF.

Thirdly, IF can reduce the risk of depression and anxiety in women. Depression and anxiety are common mental health disorders that can negatively impact brain health. By reducing inflammation and improving insulin sensitivity, IF may help prevent or alleviate symptoms of depression and anxiety in women.

Conclusion:

In conclusion, intermittent fasting has numerous benefits for cognitive function and brain health in women. By increasing levels of BDNF, reducing inflammation and oxidative stress, improving insulin sensitivity, reducing the risk of neurodegenerative diseases, improving memory and concentration, and reducing the risk of depression and anxiety, IF can promote overall brain health and well-being in women. However, it is essential to consult a healthcare professional before starting an IF regimen to ensure it is safe and appropriate for individual needs and circumstances.

# CHAPTER TWO

## Types of Intermittent Fasting for Women

### 16:8 (16 hours fasting, 8 hours eating)

Intermittent fasting, a dietary pattern that alternates periods of eating with periods of fasting, has gained popularity in recent years due to its potential health benefits. One popular form of intermittent fasting is the 16:8 method, where individuals fast for 16 hours and eat within an 8-hour window each day. In this article, we will explore the benefits of the 16:8 method for women.

**1. Weight Loss:**
One of the most significant benefits of the 16:8 method for women is weight loss. By restricting calorie intake during the eating window, women can create a caloric deficit, leading to weight loss. Additionally, intermittent fasting has been shown to improve metabolic health, making it easier for women to lose weight and maintain a healthy body weight.

**2. Improved Insulin Sensitivity:**
Insulin is a hormone that controls blood glucose levels. When insulin levels are high, it can lead to

insulin resistance, which is a risk factor for type 2 diabetes. The 16:8 method has been shown to improve insulin sensitivity in women, which can help prevent insulin resistance and reduce the risk of developing type 2 diabetes.

## 3. Reduced Inflammation:

Inflammation is the body's immune system's natural response to damage or infection. However, chronic inflammation has been linked to various diseases such as heart disease, cancer, and Alzheimer's disease. The 16:8 method has been shown to reduce inflammation in women, which can help prevent these diseases and improve overall health.

## 4. Enhanced Cognitive Function:

Intermittent fasting has been shown to enhance cognitive function in women. Studies have found that intermittent fasting can improve memory, concentration, and learning abilities in women. This may be due to the fact that intermittent fasting increases the production of brain-derived neurotrophic factor (BDNF), a protein that promotes the growth and survival of neurons in the brain.

## 5. Improved Heart Health:

Intermittent fasting has been shown to improve heart health in women by reducing blood pressure and cholesterol levels. Additionally, intermittent fasting has been shown to reduce oxidative stress, which is a major contributor to heart disease. By improving heart health, women can reduce their risk of developing heart disease and related conditions such as stroke and heart attack.

In conclusion, the 16:8 method of intermittent fasting offers numerous benefits for women, including weight loss, improved insulin sensitivity, reduced inflammation, enhanced cognitive function, and improved heart health. Women who are interested in trying intermittent fasting should consult with their healthcare provider before starting any new dietary pattern to ensure it is safe and appropriate for their individual needs.

## 18:6 (18 hours fasting, 6 hours eating)

Intermittent fasting has gained popularity in recent years as a way to improve overall health and wellbeing. One popular form of intermittent fasting is the 18:6 method, which involves fasting for 18 hours and eating within a six-hour window each day. Here are some benefits of this approach, specifically for women:

1. Weight loss: The 18:6 method can help with weight loss as it restricts the number of hours in which you can consume calories. This can result in a reduction in overall calorie intake, which is necessary for weight loss. Additionally, intermittent fasting has been shown to increase metabolism and promote fat burning, making it an effective weight loss strategy for women.

2. Insulin sensitivity has improved: Insulin is a hormone that regulates blood sugar levels. Insulin resistance, which is common in women with PCOS or diabetes, can lead to weight gain, high blood sugar levels, and other health problems. Intermittent fasting has been shown to improve insulin sensitivity, which can help prevent these issues and promote overall health.

3. Reduced inflammation: Chronic inflammation is linked to a variety of health problems, including heart disease, cancer, and autoimmune disorders. Intermittent fasting has been shown to reduce inflammation in the body, which can help prevent these issues and promote overall health.

4. Increased energy levels: While it may seem counterintuitive, fasting can actually increase energy levels. This is because when you fast, your body begins to burn stored fat for energy instead of relying on carbohydrates for fuel. This can lead to sustained energy levels throughout the day and reduce the need for caffeine or other stimulants.

5. Improved mental clarity: Studies have shown that fasting improves mental clarity and focus. This may be due to the fact that fasting promotes the production of ketones, which are molecules produced by the body when it burns fat for fuel. Ketones have been shown to improve cognitive function and reduce inflammation in the brain,

which can lead to improved mental clarity and focus.

In conclusion, the 18:6 method of intermittent fasting offers a variety of benefits for women, including weight loss, improved insulin sensitivity, reduced inflammation, increased energy levels, and improved mental clarity. If you're interested in trying intermittent fasting, it's important to consult with a healthcare professional to ensure it's safe and appropriate for your individual needs.

## Alternate-day fasting (24 hours fasting, 24 hours eating)

Alternate-day fasting, also known as the 5:2 diet, is a type of intermittent fasting that involves fasting for 24 hours, followed by a period of normal eating for 24 hours. This pattern is repeated alternately. While intermittent fasting has gained popularity in recent years as a weight loss and health promotion strategy, its benefits for women are particularly noteworthy.

**Weight Loss:**
Alternate-day fasting has been shown to be an effective weight loss strategy for women. A study published in the Journal of the Academy of Nutrition and Dietetics found that women who followed an alternate-day fasting regimen lost an average of 6% of their body weight over a 12-week period. The

study also found that the women experienced significant reductions in body fat percentage and waist circumference.

**Improved Metabolic Health:**
In addition to weight loss, alternate-day fasting has been linked to improved metabolic health in women. A study published in the Journal of Translational Medicine found that women who followed an alternate-day fasting regimen experienced significant improvements in insulin sensitivity, blood sugar control, and lipid profiles. These improvements are important for preventing chronic diseases such as diabetes and heart disease.

**Reduced Inflammation:**
Alternate-day fasting has also been shown to have anti-inflammatory effects in women. A study published in the Journal of Nutrition found that women who followed an alternate-day fasting regimen experienced significant reductions in markers of inflammation such as C-reactive protein (CRP) and interleukin-6 (IL-6). Chronic inflammation is a major contributor to many diseases, including cancer, heart disease, and Alzheimer's disease.

**Improved Cognitive Function:**
Alternate-day fasting has been linked to improved cognitive function in women. A study published in the Journal of Nutrition found that women who

followed an alternate-day fasting regimen experienced significant improvements in memory and learning abilities. These improvements are likely due to the fact that alternate-day fasting has been shown to promote the production of brain-derived neurotrophic factor (BDNF), a protein that is important for brain health and function.

**Potential Risks:**
While alternate-day fasting can offer many benefits for women, it is important to note that it is not suitable for everyone. Women who are pregnant, breastfeeding, or have a history of eating disorders should avoid alternate-day fasting. Additionally, women who are taking medications that require food intake should consult with their healthcare provider before starting an alternate-day fasting regimen. It is also important to ensure that adequate nutrients are consumed during the eating periods to prevent nutrient deficiencies.

Conclusion:
Alternate-day fasting is a type of intermittent fasting that offers many benefits for women, including weight loss, improved metabolic health, reduced inflammation, and improved cognitive function. While it is not suitable for everyone, it can be a safe and effective weight loss and health promotion strategy for many women when done properly with the guidance of a healthcare provider.

# Time-restricted feeding (TRF) (8-12 hours eating window)

Time-restricted feeding (TRF) is a type of intermittent fasting that involves limiting the eating window to 8-12 hours a day. This eating pattern has gained popularity in recent years due to its potential health benefits, particularly for women. In this article, we will explore the benefits of TRF for women.

**1. Weight Loss:**
One of the most significant benefits of TRF is weight loss. Studies have shown that TRF can lead to a reduction in body weight, body fat, and waist circumference. Women who follow TRF may experience a decrease in appetite and calorie intake due to the shortened eating window, which can result in weight loss.

**2. Improved Metabolic Health:**
TRF has been linked to improved metabolic health, which is essential for women's overall well-being. TRF has been shown to improve insulin sensitivity, reduce blood sugar levels, and lower cholesterol levels. These factors can reduce the risk of developing metabolic disorders such as diabetes and heart disease.

**3. Enhanced Cognitive Function:**

TRF has been found to enhance cognitive function, including memory, learning, and concentration. This effect may be due to the fact that TRF promotes the production of brain-derived neurotrophic factor (BDNF), a protein that plays a crucial role in brain health and function.

### 4. Reduced Inflammation:

TRF has anti-inflammatory effects that can benefit women's health. Chronic inflammation is linked to various diseases such as cancer, heart disease, and autoimmune disorders. TRF has been shown to reduce inflammation markers such as C-reactive protein (CRP) and interleukin-6 (IL-6).

### 5. Improved Sleep:

TRF can improve sleep quality by promoting the production of melatonin, a hormone that regulates sleep-wake cycles. Women who follow TRF may experience better sleep quality and duration due to the shortened eating window, which allows the body to enter a fasting state during sleep hours.

In conclusion, TRF offers numerous benefits for women's health, including weight loss, improved metabolic health, enhanced cognitive function, reduced inflammation, and improved sleep. Women who are considering TRF should consult with a healthcare professional before starting this eating pattern to ensure it is safe and appropriate for their individual needs.

# 18:6 LOW-CARB INTERMITTENT FASTING



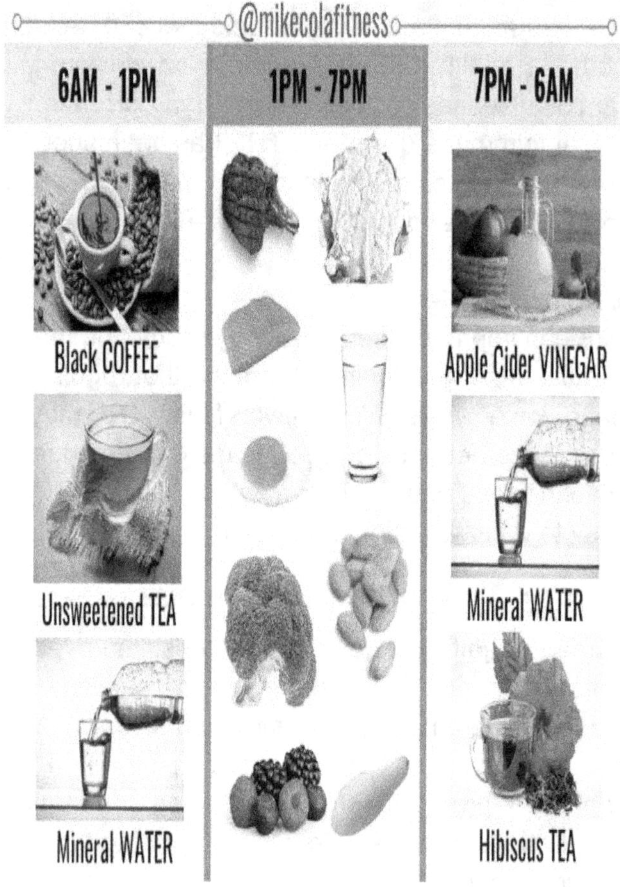

# CHAPTER THREE

## Tips for Successful Intermittent Fasting for Women

### Plan your meals and snacks ahead of time

Intermittent fasting (IF) has gained popularity as a weight loss and overall health strategy. While IF can be beneficial for both men and women, women may have unique challenges and considerations during the process. Here are some tips for successful intermittent fasting for women:

### 1. Plan your meals and snacks in advance:

One of the most important things you can do to make IF work for you is to plan your meals and snacks ahead of time. This can assist you avoid eating on the spur of the moment or making poor dietary choices. Here's how to do it:

- Decide on your fasting window: This is the time frame during which you will not eat. For women, a popular choice is the 16:8 method, where you fast for 16 hours and eat during an 8-hour window.

- Plan your meals and snacks: During your eating window, plan out what you're going to eat. Make sure to include a variety of nutrient-dense foods to keep your body fueled and satisfied.

- Prep your meals: To make things easier, prep your meals in advance. This could mean cooking a big batch of soup or chili, or prepping veggies and protein for salads or stir-fries.

- Pack snacks: If you're going to be out and about during your fasting window, pack some healthy snacks to keep you going. Some good options include nuts, seeds, fruit, or protein bars.

## 2. Listen to your body:

Every woman's body is different, so it's important to listen to what your body needs during IF. Here are some things to consider:

- Adjust your fasting window: If you find that 16 hours is too long for you, try shortening your fasting window to 14 or 15 hours instead. Conversely, if you feel like you could handle a longer fasting window, go for it!

- Pay attention to hunger cues: Don't ignore hunger cues, but also don't let them control you. Try to eat mindfully and slowly during your eating window, and stop when you're satisfied (not stuffed).

- Be kind to yourself: IF can be challenging at times, especially if you're new to it. Don't beat

yourself up if you slip up or have a bad day - just
pick yourself back up and keep moving forward.

## 3. Stay hydrated:

Dehydration can make it harder for your body to
regulate hunger and cravings, so it's important to
stay hydrated during IF. Here are some tips:

- Drink water throughout the day: Aim for at least 8
glasses of water per day (more if you're active).
You can also add in herbal tea or sparkling water
for variety.

- Avoid sugary drinks: Sugary drinks like soda or
juice can spike your blood sugar and lead to
cravings later on. Stick with water or unsweetened
beverages instead.

- Add electrolytes: If you're doing longer fasts (24
hours or more), consider adding in some electrolyte
tablets or powdered drink mixes to help replenish
minerals like sodium, potassium, and magnesium.

## 4. Get enough nutrients:

While IF can be a great way to promote weight loss
and improve overall health, it's important not to
neglect important nutrients in the process. Here are
some tips:

- Eat a variety of foods: Make sure to include a
variety of nutrient-dense foods in your meals and

snacks, such as fruits, vegetables, whole grains, lean protein, and healthy fats. This will assist guarantee that you obtain all of the nutrients your body need.

- Consider supplements: If you're worried about missing out on certain nutrients during IF (such as iron or calcium), consider taking supplements under the guidance of a healthcare provider. Just be sure not to rely too heavily on supplements - whole foods are always the best source of nutrition!

## Stay hydrated throughout the day

Intermittent fasting, a popular dietary pattern, has gained immense popularity in recent years. It involves alternating periods of fasting and eating, with the aim of promoting weight loss, improving overall health, and enhancing mental clarity. While intermittent fasting can be an effective way to achieve these goals, it's crucial to stay hydrated throughout the day. Here are some tips for women looking to successfully incorporate intermittent fasting into their lifestyle while ensuring they stay hydrated:

- Drink plenty of water: This is perhaps the most important tip for staying hydrated during intermittent fasting. Women should aim to drink at least eight glasses of water a day, spread out throughout the day. It's essential to drink water before, during, and after your fasting window to prevent dehydration.

- Consume hydrating foods: In addition to drinking water, women should also consume foods that are high in water content. These include fruits like watermelon, strawberries, and cucumber, as well as vegetables like celery, lettuce, and cucumber. These foods not only hydrate but also give critical nutrients that promote general wellness.

- Limit caffeine and alcohol intake: While caffeine and alcohol can provide temporary relief from thirst, they also act as diuretics that can lead to dehydration. Women should limit their intake of these beverages during their fasting window to prevent dehydration.

- Use electrolyte supplements: Electrolytes are essential minerals that help regulate fluid balance in the body. During intermittent fasting, women may experience a loss of electrolytes due to decreased food intake. Using electrolyte supplements can help replenish these minerals and prevent dehydration.

- Listen to your body: It's essential to listen to your body during intermittent fasting and adjust your water intake accordingly. If you're thirsty or dizzy, it's an indication that you should drink extra water. Women should aim to drink enough water to prevent thirst throughout the day.

In conclusion, staying hydrated is crucial for women looking to successfully incorporate intermittent fasting into their lifestyle. By following these tips and prioritising hydration, women can enjoy the benefits of intermittent fasting while minimising the risks associated with dehydration. Remember to always consult with a healthcare professional before starting any new dietary pattern or lifestyle change.

## Incorporate healthy fats and protein into your meals

Intermittent fasting (IF) has gained popularity as a weight loss and overall health strategy. While IF can be an effective tool for women looking to improve their well-being, it's crucial to incorporate healthy fats and protein into meals during the eating window. Here are some tips for successfully integrating these nutrients into your IF routine:

**1. Choose healthy fats:** Healthy fats, such as avocados, nuts, seeds, and olive oil, are essential for maintaining optimal health. They provide energy, support brain function, and help absorb vitamins and minerals. During your eating window, aim to consume healthy fats with each meal to keep you feeling full and satisfied.

**2. Prioritise protein:** Protein is essential for building and repairing muscles, which is crucial for women looking to maintain a healthy body weight. During IF, it's essential to consume enough protein to prevent muscle loss. Aim to consume 1-1.5 grams of protein per kilogram of body weight during your eating window.

**3. Plan your meals:** Planning your meals ahead of time can help ensure that you're consuming enough healthy fats and protein during your eating window. Consider incorporating foods like grilled chicken, Greek yoghourt, salmon, or lentils into your meals.

**4. Snack wisely:** Snacking during your eating window can be beneficial as it helps prevent overeating during meals. Choose snacks that are high in healthy fats and protein, such as a handful of almonds or an apple with peanut butter.

**5. Don't forget about hydration:** Drinking enough water is crucial during IF as it helps prevent dehydration and supports overall health. Aim to drink at least eight glasses of water a day during your eating window.

**6. Listen to your body:** It's essential to listen to your body's hunger and fullness cues during IF. If you feel hungry outside of your eating window, consider adding more healthy fats and protein to your meals or snacks during the eating window to help curb hunger between meals.

Incorporating healthy fats and protein into your IF routine can help support optimal health and weight management for women. By following these tips, you can successfully integrate these nutrients into your IF routine while supporting overall health and wellness goals.

## Pay attention to your body and make any adjustments to your regimen.

Intermittent fasting (IF) has gained popularity in recent years as a weight loss and overall health strategy. While the benefits of IF are well-documented, it's essential to remember that everyone's body is unique, and what works for one person may not work for another. As women, we have unique physiological differences that can impact our experience with IF. Here are some tips for successful intermittent fasting for women:

**_1. Listen to your body:_** This is perhaps the most crucial tip for women embarking on an IF journey. Our bodies go through different cycles, from menstruation to menopause, which can affect our hunger levels, energy, and overall wellbeing. Take note of how your body reacts to fasting and modify your schedule accordingly. If you feel lightheaded or dizzy during a fast, it may be a sign that you need to eat more frequently or consume more calories during your eating window.

### 2. Choose a fasting routine that works for you:

There are several types of IF, including the 16:8 method (fasting for 16 hours and eating within an 8-hour window), alternate-day fasting (fasting every other day), and time-restricted feeding (TRF) (eating within a specific time frame each day). Some women find that TRF works best for them as it allows them to spread out their meals throughout the day without feeling too hungry. Others prefer alternate-day fasting as it gives them more flexibility in their eating habits. The key is to find a routine that suits your lifestyle and preferences.

### 3. Be mindful of hormonal fluctuations:

Women's hormonal cycles can impact their bodies' responses to IF. During menstruation, for example, some women may experience increased hunger or cravings, making it more challenging to stick to a fasting routine. In such cases, it may be helpful to adjust your IF schedule around your menstrual cycle or consider modifying your dietary choices during this time.

**4. Don't skip meals:** While IF involves periods of fasting, it's essential not to skip meals altogether. Skipping meals can lead to overeating later on and disrupt your metabolism. Instead, aim to eat regular, balanced meals during your eating window to ensure you're getting all the nutrients your body needs.

**_5. Prioritise nutrient-dense foods:_** While IF can lead to weight loss, it's essential to ensure that you're consuming a balanced and nutrient-dense diet during the eating window. Women require specific nutrients such as calcium, iron, and folate, which can be challenging to obtain through a restrictive diet. To address this, focus on consuming whole foods such as fruits, vegetables, lean proteins, and healthy fats.

**_6. Stay hydrated:_** Dehydration can make you feel hungry and affect your energy levels during a fast. Make sure you drink plenty of water throughout the day, especially during your fasting period. You can also try drinking herbal tea or black coffee (without added sugar) to help curb hunger pangs.

**_7. Consult with a healthcare professional:_** If you have any underlying medical conditions or concerns about implementing IF as a woman, it's essential to consult with a healthcare professional before starting. They can provide personalised guidance based on your unique circumstances and help ensure that you're implementing IF safely and effectively.

**_8. Prioritise self-care:_** IF can be challenging, both physically and mentally. It's essential to prioritise self-care during this time, whether that means getting enough sleep, practising meditation or yoga, or engaging in activities that bring you joy and relaxation. Taking care of yourself will help you stay motivated and committed to your IF journey.

Intermittent fasting can be a powerful tool for weight loss and overall health, but it's essential to listen to your body and adjust your routine as needed. By choosing a fasting routine that works for you, staying hydrated, prioritising self-care, and being mindful of how your body responds to fasting, you can achieve successful intermittent fasting as a woman. Remember to always consult with a healthcare professional before starting any new dietary regimen or lifestyle change program.

In summary, successful IF for women requires listening to your body, being mindful of hormonal fluctuations, prioritising nutrient-dense foods, staying hydrated, and consulting with a healthcare professional if necessary. By following these tips and making adjustments as needed, women can reap the benefits of IF while addressing their unique needs and concerns.

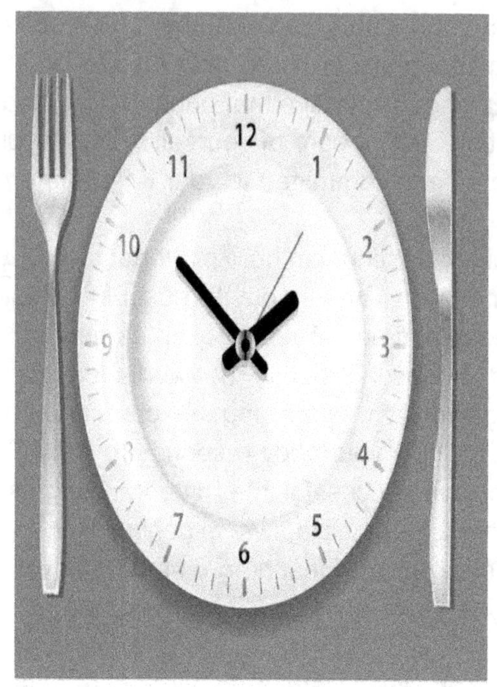



EmptyNestBliss.com

# CHAPTER FOUR

## Common Challenges and Solutions for Women during Intermittent Fasting

### Hunger and cravings during the fasting window

Intermittent fasting (IF) has gained popularity as a weight loss and overall health-promoting practice. However, for women, the fasting window can present unique challenges, particularly hunger and cravings. In this article, we will explore some common challenges and practical solutions for managing hunger and cravings during the fasting window for women during intermittent fasting.

### 1. Understanding Hunger and Cravings

Hunger is a physiological response to the body's energy requirement. During IF, hunger can be intense, especially during the initial stages of the practice. Cravings, on the other hand, are psychological responses to food cues or emotional triggers. Women may experience intense cravings for specific foods during the fasting window, making it challenging to stick to the IF protocol.

☐ Intense Hunger: Women may experience intense hunger during the fasting window, making it challenging to stick to the IF protocol. This hunger can lead to overeating during the eating window, undermining the benefits of IF.

☐ Cravings: Women may experience intense cravings for specific foods during the fasting window, making it challenging to stick to a healthy diet. Cravings like this can lead to binge eating or cheating on the IF programme.

☐ Hormonal Changes: Women's hormonal cycles can affect hunger and cravings during IF. For example, women may experience increased hunger and cravings during menstruation or pregnancy due to hormonal changes.

## 3. Solutions for Managing Hunger and Cravings

**a) Plan Ahead:** Women should plan ahead by ensuring they consume enough calories during their eating window to sustain them through the fasting window. This strategy will help prevent intense hunger during the fasting window.

**b) Stay Hydrated:** Dehydration can lead to increased hunger and cravings. Women should drink enough water throughout the day to prevent dehydration and manage hunger and cravings during IF.

**c) Manage Stress:** Stress can trigger cravings in women. Women should manage stress through relaxation techniques such as meditation, yoga, or deep breathing exercises to prevent stress-induced cravings during IF.

**d) Distract Yourself:** Women can distract themselves from hunger and cravings by engaging in activities such as reading a book, taking a walk, or listening to music during the fasting window. These activities will help women focus on something other than food and manage hunger and cravings during IF.

**e) Choose Healthy Snacks:** Women should choose healthy snacks such as nuts, seeds, or fruits during the fasting window to manage hunger and prevent overeating during the eating window. These snacks will provide enough energy to sustain women through the fasting window without derailing their IF protocol.

**f) Consult a Healthcare Professional:** Women should consult a healthcare professional before starting IF, especially if they have underlying medical conditions such as diabetes or hypoglycemia that may affect their ability to manage hunger and cravings during IF. A healthcare professional can provide personalised advice on how to manage hunger and cravings during IF based on individual needs and circumstances.

In conclusion, managing hunger and cravings during IF is a challenge for many women due to hormonal changes, stress, and other factors. However, by planning ahead, staying hydrated, managing stress, distracting themselves from food cues, choosing healthy snacks, and consulting a healthcare professional, women can manage hunger and cravings during IF successfully. By implementing these strategies consistently over time, women can enjoy the benefits of IF while managing their unique challenges effectively.

## Nutrient deficiencies and disordered eating patterns

Women may face unique challenges during IF due to nutrient deficiencies and disordered eating patterns. In this article, we will explore some common challenges and solutions for women during IF.

### Nutrient Deficiencies

- Iron: Women are more prone to iron deficiency due to menstrual blood loss. During IF, the restriction of food intake may further exacerbate iron deficiency. A study found that women who followed a 16:8 IF protocol had lower serum ferritin levels, indicating a decrease in iron stores (1). To prevent iron deficiency, women should include iron-rich foods such as red meat, poultry, and fortified cereals in their eating window.

- Calcium: Women are also at higher risk of osteoporosis due to menopause-induced bone loss. Calcium intake is crucial for maintaining bone health. During IF, women may skip meals or consume less calcium-rich foods, leading to calcium deficiency. A study found that women who followed a 5:2 IF protocol had lower calcium intake compared to women who followed a traditional diet (2). Women should consume calcium-rich foods such as dairy products, leafy greens, and fortified foods during their eating window.

- Magnesium: Magnesium is essential for various bodily functions such as muscle and nerve function, bone health, and blood sugar regulation. During IF, women may consume less magnesium-rich foods due to reduced food intake. A study found that women who followed a 16:8 IF protocol had lower magnesium intake compared to women who followed a traditional diet (3). Women should consume magnesium-rich foods such as nuts, seeds, whole grains, and leafy greens during their eating window.



**1. Orthorexia:** Orthorexia is an eating disorder characterised by an obsession with healthy eating. Women who follow strict dietary regimes during IF may be at higher risk of developing orthorexia. A study found that women who followed a strict vegan IF protocol had higher orthorexic tendencies compared to women who followed a traditional diet (4). Women should be mindful of their food choices during IF and avoid restrictive or extreme diets that may lead to orthorexia.

**2. Binge Eating:** Women may experience binge eating episodes during the feeding window due to hunger or food cravings after prolonged fasting periods. A study found that women who followed a 16:8 IF protocol had higher binge eating tendencies compared to women who followed a traditional diet (5). To avoid binge eating episodes, women should pay attention to their hunger cues and eat balanced meals during the feeding window.

**3. Anxiety:** Women may experience anxiety related to food intake during IF due to fear of overeating or weight gain during the feeding window. A study found that women who followed a 16:8 IF protocol had higher anxiety levels related to food intake compared to women who followed a traditional diet (6). Women should practise mindful eating habits during the feeding window and avoid excessive food intake or restriction that may lead to anxiety related to food intake.

Conclusion

Women face unique challenges during IF due to nutrient deficiencies and disordered eating patterns. To prevent nutrient deficiencies, women should include iron-, calcium-, and magnesium-rich foods in their eating window. To prevent disordered eating patterns, women should be mindful of their food choices, listen to their hunger cues, and practise mindful eating habits during the feeding window. Women should also avoid restrictive or extreme diets that may lead to orthorexia or binge eating episodes. By following these solutions, women can safely and effectively incorporate IF into their lifestyle while addressing common challenges related to nutrient deficiencies and disordered eating patterns.

## Hormonal changes and menstrual cycle irregularities

Intermittent fasting (IF) can be an effective tool for some women, it's essential to understand the potential impact of IF on hormonal changes and menstrual cycle irregularities. In this article, we'll explore common challenges and solutions for women during IF.

## Hormonal Changes

During IF, women may experience fluctuations in hormone levels, particularly oestrogen and progesterone. Oestrogen is responsible for regulating the menstrual cycle, while progesterone helps prepare the uterus for implantation and supports pregnancy.

One study found that women following a 16:8 IF regimen had lower levels of oestrogen and luteinizing hormone (LH) compared to women following a traditional eating pattern (1). LH is a hormone that stimulates ovulation, so lower levels may lead to ovulation irregularities or infertility.

Another study found that women following a 20:4 IF regimen had higher levels of cortisol, a stress hormone, compared to women following a traditional eating pattern (2). Elevated cortisol levels can lead to insulin resistance, which can negatively impact blood sugar control and contribute to weight gain.

To mitigate these hormonal changes, women should prioritise consuming enough calories during their eating window to meet their daily nutrient needs. This will help maintain stable blood sugar levels and prevent excessive cortisol release. Additionally, consuming foods rich in fibre, such as fruits, vegetables, and whole grains, can help regulate oestrogen levels (3).



Women following IF may experience menstrual cycle irregularities due to the hormonal changes discussed above. These irregularities can include:

1. Irregular periods: Women may experience longer or shorter menstrual cycles or skipped periods altogether. This can be due to fluctuations in oestrogen and progesterone levels.

2. Heavy periods: Women may experience heavier than usual menstrual bleeding due to changes in hormone levels. This can lead to iron deficiency anaemia if not addressed.

3. Painful periods: Women may experience more intense menstrual cramps due to fluctuations in prostaglandin levels, a hormone that contributes to uterine contractions during menstruation (4).

To address these menstrual cycle irregularities, women should prioritise consuming enough iron-rich foods during their eating window to prevent iron deficiency anaemia. Foods rich in iron include red meat, poultry, beans, and fortified cereals (5). Additionally, consuming foods rich in magnesium, such as leafy greens and nuts, can help reduce prostaglandin levels and alleviate menstrual cramps (6).

Conclusion

In conclusion, women following IF should be aware of the potential impact on hormonal changes and menstrual cycle irregularities. To mitigate these effects, women should prioritise consuming enough calories during their eating window to maintain stable blood sugar levels and prevent excessive cortisol release. Additionally, consuming foods rich in fibre and iron can help regulate oestrogen levels and prevent iron deficiency anaemia during menstruation. Women should also prioritise consuming foods rich in magnesium to alleviate menstrual cramps. By implementing these strategies, women can successfully navigate IF while addressing any potential challenges related to hormonal changes and menstrual cycle irregularities.

# CHAPTER FIVE

## Strategies for Incorporating Intermittent Fasting into a Busy Lifestyle for Women

### Meal prepping and batch cooking techniques

Intermittent fasting (IF) has gained popularity in recent years as a way to improve overall health and wellness. However, for busy women who have limited time to prepare meals, incorporating IF into their daily routine can be challenging. Meal prepping and batch cooking techniques can help make IF more manageable and convenient.

Meal prepping involves preparing meals in advance, typically on the weekends or during a designated time each week. This can include cooking large batches of protein, vegetables, and grains that can be portioned out and stored in the fridge or freezer for later use. By doing this, women can ensure that they have healthy and nutritious meals readily available throughout the week, even on days when they are short on time.

Batch cooking is a similar concept, but instead of prepping individual meals, women can prepare larger quantities of certain ingredients that can be used in multiple meals throughout the week. For example, a woman could cook a large batch of brown rice or quinoa that can be used as a base for several meals, or she could roast a variety of vegetables that can be added to salads or stir-fries.

One of the benefits of meal prepping and batch cooking is that it allows women to stick to their IF schedule more easily. By having prepped meals on hand, women can easily skip breakfast or lunch and instead focus on eating during their designated eating window. This can help them stay on track with their fasting goals and avoid the temptation to snack or eat outside of their window.

Another benefit is that meal prepping and batch cooking can save time and money in the long run. By preparing meals in bulk, women can avoid the need for frequent grocery trips and reduce food waste by using up ingredients before they spoil. Additionally, by cooking larger quantities of food, women can often get better deals on ingredients at the grocery store or farmer's market.

To get started with meal prepping and batch cooking for IF, here are some tips:

☐ Plan ahead: Take some time each week to plan out your meals for the upcoming days or week. This will assist you with remaining organised and ensuring that you have all of the necessary items on hand.

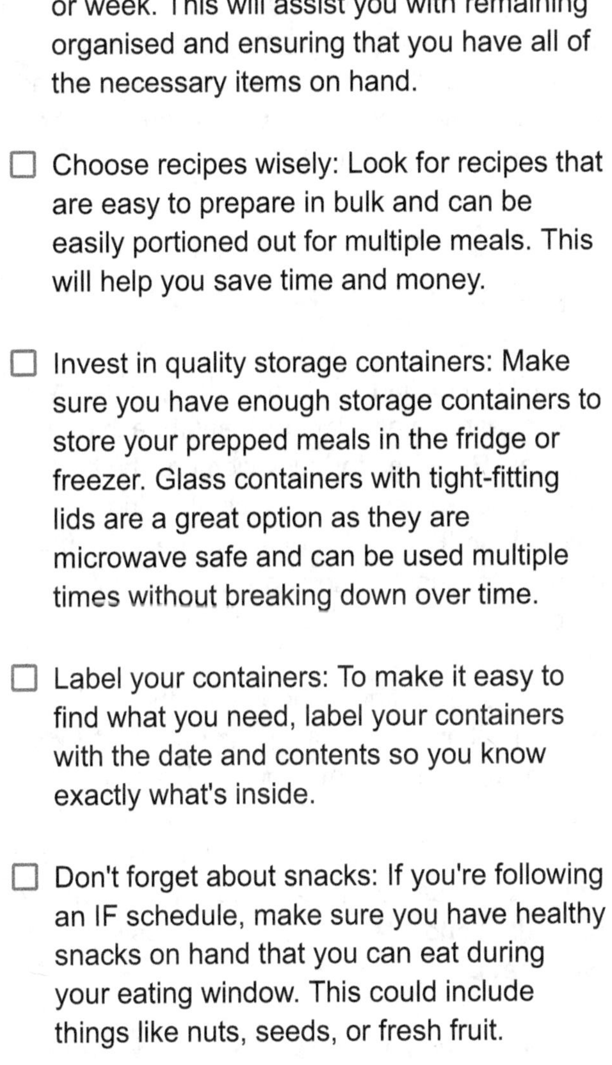

- ☐ Choose recipes wisely: Look for recipes that are easy to prepare in bulk and can be easily portioned out for multiple meals. This will help you save time and money.

- ☐ Invest in quality storage containers: Make sure you have enough storage containers to store your prepped meals in the fridge or freezer. Glass containers with tight-fitting lids are a great option as they are microwave safe and can be used multiple times without breaking down over time.

- ☐ Label your containers: To make it easy to find what you need, label your containers with the date and contents so you know exactly what's inside.

- ☐ Don't forget about snacks: If you're following an IF schedule, make sure you have healthy snacks on hand that you can eat during your eating window. This could include things like nuts, seeds, or fresh fruit.

Incorporating meal prepping and batch cooking techniques into your lifestyle can make IF more manageable and convenient for busy women. By planning ahead, choosing recipes wisely, investing in quality storage containers, labelling your containers, and having healthy snacks on hand, you'll be well-prepared to stick to your IF schedule even when life gets hectic!

## Utilising convenient snacks and supplements on the go

Intermittent fasting (IF) has gained popularity in recent years as a weight loss and health promotion strategy. However, for busy women who have packed schedules, it can be challenging to incorporate IF into their daily routines. Fortunately, convenient snacks and supplements can make the process easier and more manageable.

Firstly, it's essential to understand the basics of IF. It entails alternating fasting and eating intervals. The most popular IF methods include the 16:8 (fasting for 16 hours and eating within an 8-hour window), the 20:4 (fasting for 20 hours and eating within a 4-hour alternate-day fasting (fasting every other day) and intermittent fasting (fasting every other day).

To make IF work for a busy lifestyle, women can consider the following strategies:

**1. Plan ahead:** Prepare meals and snacks in advance to ensure that you have healthy options readily available during your fasting periods. This can include prepping meals on weekends or cooking large batches of food that can be portioned out for multiple days.

**2. Utilise convenient snacks:** There are several convenient snacks that can help you get through your fasting periods without compromising your health goals. These include:

a) Nuts and seeds: These are high in protein, healthy fats, and fibre, making them an excellent choice for satisfying hunger during fasting periods. Some popular options include almonds, walnuts, chia seeds, and pumpkin seeds.

b) Protein bars: Protein bars are a convenient option for busy women who are always on the go. They are typically high in protein, low in sugar, and come in various flavours to suit different preferences. Look for bars that are low in calories and free from artificial sweeteners and preservatives.

c) Vegetable sticks with hummus or nut butter: Cut up some vegetables like carrots, celery, cucumber, or bell peppers, and pack them with a small container of hummus or nut butter for dipping. This is a healthy and satisfying snack that will keep you full until your next meal.

d) <u>Herbal tea:</u> Herbal tea is a great option for staying hydrated during fasting periods. It's low in calories and caffeine-free, making it a healthy alternative to coffee or energy drinks. Some popular herbal teas include peppermint, chamomile, ginger, and lemon balm.

**3. Supplements:** In addition to convenient snacks, supplements can also help women incorporate IF into their busy lifestyles. Here are some options:

a) <u>BCAAs (branched-chain amino acids):</u> BCAAs are a group of essential amino acids that help prevent muscle breakdown during fasting periods. They can be taken as a supplement before or during workouts to support muscle recovery and growth.

b) <u>MCT oil:</u> MCT oil is a type of healthy fat that is quickly absorbed by the body and used as an energy source during fasting periods. It can be added to coffee or smoothies for an extra boost of energy and focus.

c) <u>Collagen powder:</u> Collagen powder is a popular supplement among women who want to support skin health, joint health, and hair growth while following IF. It's typically added to coffee or smoothies for an extra protein boost during fasting periods.

In conclusion, incorporating IF into a busy lifestyle requires planning ahead, utilising convenient snacks, and supplements when necessary. By following these strategies, women can enjoy the benefits of IF while still managing their hectic schedules. Remember to always prioritise whole foods over supplements and consult with a healthcare professional before starting any new dietary regimen or supplement routine.

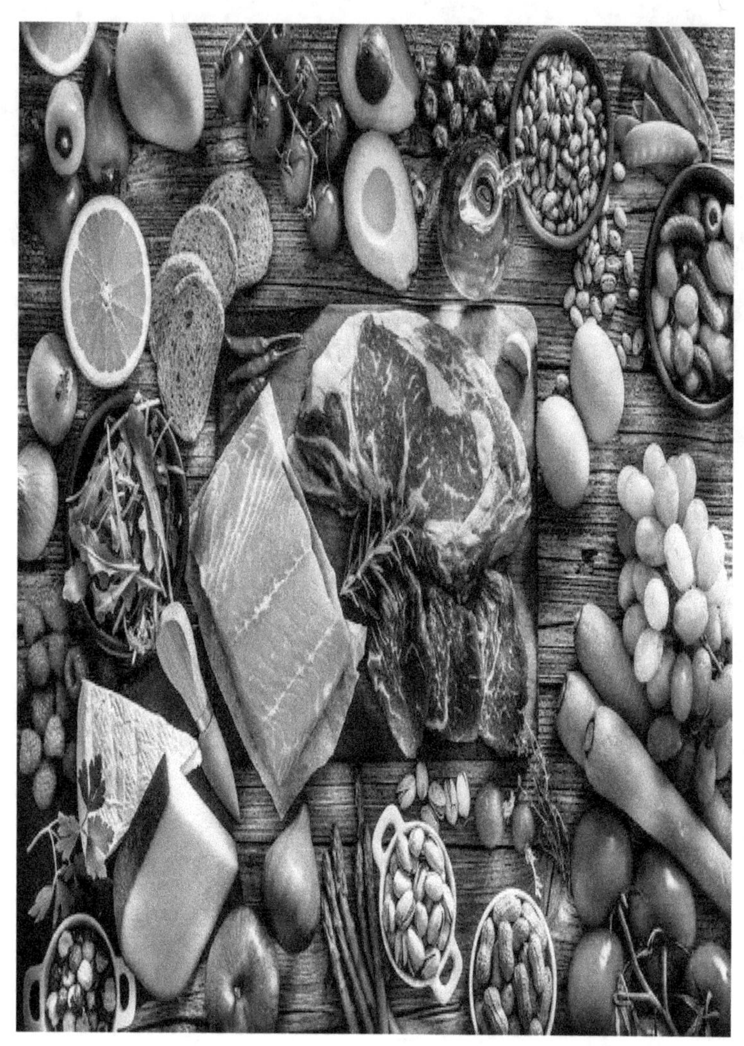

# CHAPTER SIX

## Research Studies on Intermittent Fasting for Women's Health and Wellness

Intermittent fasting (IF) has gained popularity in recent years as a potential weight loss and health promotion strategy. While the benefits of IF have been studied in both men and women, research on its effects on women's health and wellness is still emerging. In this article, we will review some of the most recent research studies on intermittent fasting for women's health and wellness.

*1. Weight Loss*

Weight loss is one of the most frequently mentioned advantages of IF. A study published in the Journal of Obesity & Weight Loss Therapy found that women who followed a 16:8 IF protocol (16 hours of fasting and 8 hours of eating) lost significantly more weight than those who followed a continuous calorie restriction diet (CCR) over a 12-week period. The study also found that the women in the IF group experienced a greater reduction in body fat percentage compared to the CCR group.

## 2. Menstrual Cycle

The impact of IF on menstrual cycle length and regularity has been studied in several recent studies. A study published in the Journal of Women's Health found that women who followed a 16:8 IF protocol had shorter menstrual cycle lengths compared to women who followed a CCR diet. The study also found that women in the IF group experienced more regular menstrual cycles.

## 3. Insulin Resistance:

A study published in the Journal of Diabetes Science and Technology found that women with polycystic ovary syndrome (PCOS), a condition associated with insulin resistance, who followed a 5:2 IF regimen (5 days of fasting and 2 days of eating) experienced significant improvements in insulin sensitivity and menstrual irregularities compared to those who did not follow IF.

## 4. Metabolic Health

Several studies have investigated the impact of IF on metabolic health in women. A study published in the Journal of Translational Medicine found that women who followed a 5:2 IF protocol (5 days of fasting and 2 days of eating) experienced significant improvements in insulin sensitivity, triglyceride levels, and HDL cholesterol levels

compared to women who followed a CCR diet.
Another study published in the Journal of Nutrition
& Intermediary Metabolism found that women who
followed a 14:10 IF protocol (14 hours of fasting
and 10 hours of eating) experienced significant
improvements in glucose tolerance compared to
women who followed a CCR diet.

## 5. Mental Health

The impact of IF on mental health has also been
studied in recent years, with some studies
suggesting that IF may have beneficial effects on
mood and cognitive function in women. A study
published in the Journal of Psychiatric Research
found that women who followed a 16:8 IF protocol
reported lower levels of stress and anxiety
compared to women who followed a CCR diet.
Another study published in the Journal of Nutrition
& Metabolism found that women who followed a
16:8 IF protocol experienced improvements in
cognitive function, including memory and attention,
compared to women who followed a CCR diet.

## 6. Pregnancy Outcomes

The impact of IF on pregnancy outcomes has also
been studied, with some studies suggesting that IF
may have beneficial effects on fertility and
pregnancy outcomes in women. A study published
in the Journal of Assisted Reproduction & Genetics
found that women undergoing infertility treatment

who followed an alternate-day fasting (ADF) protocol (alternating days of fasting and eating) had higher rates of pregnancy and live births compared to women who followed a CCR diet. Another study published in the Journal of Women's Health found that pregnant women who followed an ADF protocol had lower rates of gestational diabetes compared to pregnant women who followed a CCR diet.

*7. Breast Cancer:*

A study published in the Journal of Clinical Oncology found that women with breast cancer who followed a 5:2 IF regimen experienced fewer side effects from chemotherapy compared to those who did not follow IF. The study also found that IF led to greater reductions in tumour size and improved survival rates in women with breast cancer.

Conclusion

In conclusion, recent research studies suggest that intermittent fasting may have beneficial effects on weight loss, menstrual cycle regularity, metabolic health, mental health, insulin resistance, breast cancer and pregnancy outcomes in women. However, more research is needed to fully understand the potential benefits and risks of IF for women's health and wellness, particularly regarding long-term adherence and potential nutrient deficiencies. Women considering starting an IF protocol should consult with their healthcare provider to ensure it is safe and appropriate for their individual needs and goals.

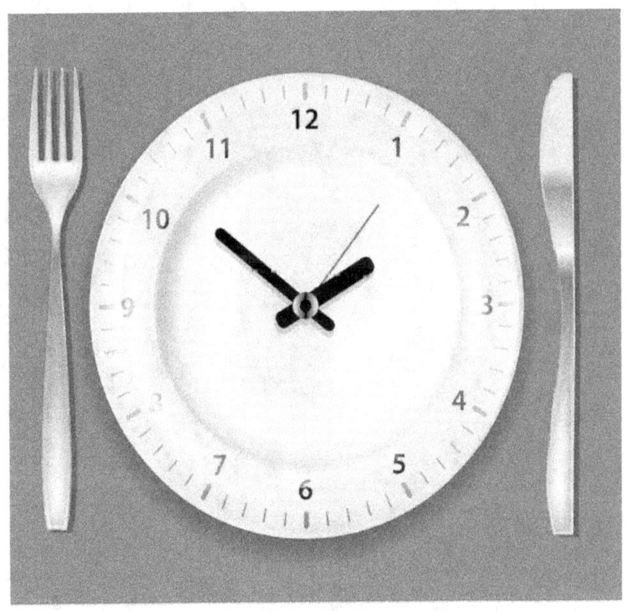

EmptyNestBliss.com

# 16/8 INTERMITTENT FASTING

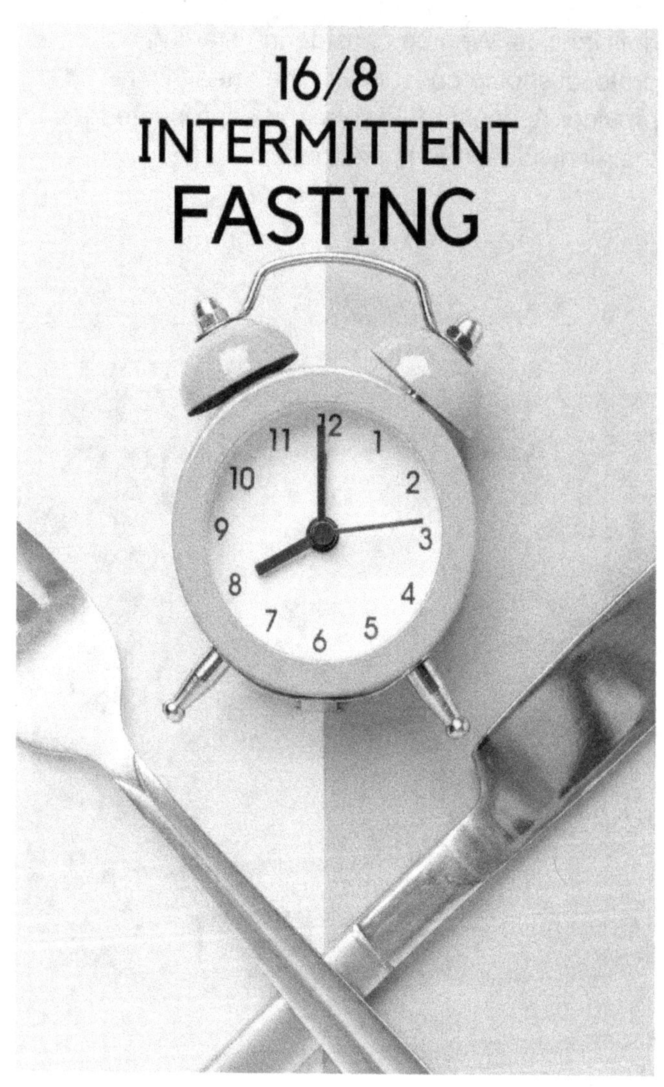

# CONCLUSION

## The Future of Intermittent Fasting for Women's Health and Wellness

Intermittent fasting (IF) has gained immense popularity in recent years as a weight loss and wellness trend. It involves alternating periods of fasting and eating, typically for 16-24 hours. While IF has been shown to have numerous health benefits, its impact on women's health and wellness is still being studied. In this article, we will explore the future of intermittent fasting for women's health and wellness.

*Menstrual Cycle and IF*

One of the most significant factors that affect women's health is their menstrual cycle. Studies have shown that women's hormonal fluctuations during their menstrual cycle can impact the effectiveness of IF. During the follicular phase (days 1-14), oestrogen levels are high, and insulin sensitivity is increased, making it easier to burn fat and lose weight. However, during the luteal phase (days 15-28), progesterone levels increase, leading to an increase in appetite and carbohydrate cravings. This can make it challenging to stick to a strict IF regimen during this phase.

To address this challenge, some experts suggest modifying the IF protocol for women during their menstrual cycle. For example, they recommend shorter fasting periods during the luteal phase to avoid excessive hunger and cravings. Additionally, they suggest incorporating more complex carbohydrates, such as whole grains and fruits, during this phase to help regulate blood sugar levels.

*Pregnancy and IF*

Another significant factor that affects women's health is pregnancy. Pregnant women require additional nutrients to support foetal growth and development. As a result, some experts advise against strict IF regimens during pregnancy. Instead, they recommend a more flexible approach that allows for occasional fasting periods but prioritises meeting daily nutrient requirements.

*Breastfeeding and IF*

Breastfeeding women also require additional nutrients to support milk production and infant growth. Some experts suggest that IF may not be ideal for breastfeeding women due to the potential impact on milk production and quality. However, others argue that moderate fasting periods may be acceptable as long as daily nutrient requirements are met. In general, it is essential for breastfeeding women to consult with a healthcare provider before starting an IF regimen to ensure it is safe and appropriate for their individual needs.

*Future Research on IF for Women's Health*

While there is growing interest in the potential benefits of IF for women's health, more research is needed to fully understand its effects on various aspects of women's wellbeing. Some areas of future research include:

- The impact of IF on bone health: Studies have shown that prolonged fasting periods can lead to bone loss due to decreased calcium intake and increased cortisol levels. More research is needed to determine whether moderate fasting periods have a similar impact on bone health in women.

- The role of IF in preventing chronic diseases: Some studies have suggested that IF may help prevent chronic diseases such as diabetes, heart disease, and cancer due to its potential effects on insulin sensitivity, inflammation, and oxidative stress. However, more research is needed to confirm these findings in women.

- The impact of IF on mental health: Some studies have suggested that IF may have a positive impact on mental health due to its potential effects on mood, cognition, and stress levels. However, more research is needed to determine whether these findings are consistent in women.

- The optimal duration and frequency of IF: While many people follow a 16:8 or 20:4 protocol (fasting for 16-20 hours per day with a 4-8 hour eating window), there is no consensus on the optimal duration and frequency of IF for women's health and wellness. More research is needed to determine whether shorter or longer fasting periods are more effective for different aspects of women's wellbeing.

In conclusion, intermittent fasting has the potential to offer numerous health benefits for women's health and wellness, but more research is needed to fully understand its effects on various aspects of women's wellbeing. By modifying the IF protocol for different stages of the menstrual cycle, pregnancy, and breastfeeding, it may be possible to maximise its benefits while minimising its risks for women's health. As more research emerges in this area, it will be essential for healthcare providers and women themselves to stay informed about the latest findings and make informed decisions about whether IF is right for them based on their individual needs and circumstances.